FACE YOGA
Natural face lifting in just 14 days

JOAN CARTER

Copyright © 2013 Joan Carter

All rights reserved.

ISBN: **1484938291**
ISBN-13: 978-1484938294

DEDICATION

This book is dedicated to my daughter Lucia who is more wise than I've ever been, to my great dear friend Marija Jukic Zubak for being tremendous support and my cousin Ruth Guglielmi for advice and support! Girls this one is for you!

CONTENTS

	Acknowledgments	i
1	Introduction	1
2	What is face yoga	3
3	The eyes	6
4	Face and neck exercises	20
5	Work out	30
	About the Author	

ACKNOWLEDGMENTS

I would like to thank my family, my daughter and husband, for believing in me and my path while creating my books.
Also my great friends Maria, Ruth and Lea for being my support and encouragement when I needed it most!
Thank you Azra, my beautiful and cooperative model for being open and positive and also for being so professional!
Also many thanks to CreateSpace for giving opportunities to many authors to express ideas and creativity, without you none of this would be possible!

1 INTRODUCTION

There is no doubt any more that the media is forming our opinion on absolutely everything. It's not easy to be a women in such a world. What is beauty? Photoshoped, anorexic, unhealthy looking models? Or maybe botoxed, filled with silicone, aging stars, who can't even smile after all that surgery? They pull out their ribs, take out healthy teeth and replace them with artificial ones, take hormone shots to stay slim. Where does it all end? The most damaging fact of all is that generations of girls and young women feel ugly and unwanted when they compare themselves to these fake people who have barely a few original parts left in their bodies! The fashion and beauty industry deliberately ruined generations of women, their natural confidence and self –respect, so they can sell them all of those products they don't actually need and which won't make them look like these "fake" women they look up to. Do you remember the stars from 60', 70' and even part of the 80's? Those girls were really beautiful, worked out and really gave their best to look sexy and attractive, no matter how old they were.

There is a way to be beautiful without plastic surgery,

without pulling out your ribs and sticking needles in your face. It's eating healthy, practicing sports, yoga and face yoga. This is not a new thing! It was out there for thousands of years, just waiting to be thought and used again. Face yoga is a craft where you practice muscles of your face, that eventually pull your skin and make your face look younger and healthier. If you combine this practice with regular yoga the benefits are even greater. So I'm going to show you how easy and quickly you can reach visible results and look younger in two weeks. As you continue with exercises, the results will be even more visible and lasting. The practice itself doesn't take much time, not more than 10 minutes a day. If you want to progress faster you can exercise up to 30 minutes a day and enjoy the wonderful results of your effort. In this program I included also some affirmation and visualization exercises, than can really add up to a satisfying end result as the psychological aspect of the development is vital.

I wish you persistence and a wonderful journey with this booklet, so that you can truly enjoy the beauty and the diva that you really are!

The Author

2 WHAT IS FACE YOGA

Beauty is eternity gazing at itself in a mirror. ~ Kahlil Gibran

Let's start by making it clear what Face Yoga is about. When you look at the exercises it may look like a massage or a funny face contest, but we actually do is stimulate muscles in your face area to give them back the firmness and strength they once had. They should be treated like all the other muscles in the body, but do you really think about them when you go to the gym? Or take a Pilates class? Well, no one does! There are so many products advertised to give you a face lifting or a "new shine", but nothing can really do that because all these things work on surface level!
Your muscles must be exercised and toned to grow and give your face a firm and younger look.
The Face Yoga exercises are very simple and may even look as if they are too simple to work. But I learned a long time ago that best solutions come to me in simple forms! With Face Yoga not only will your muscles be firmer, blood and oxygen will "flow" more freely and give your skin the much needed nutrients. So if you practice those exercises daily

there will be many benefits and they will come very quickly too. People are really into the "quick fix solution" and that is the number one reason why plastic surgery is so popular. But it's damaging too and after a while the results are not that good any more. Face Yoga is also a quick solution and can give you so much benefit if you practice it daily. Relaxation will also be one of the benefits of regular training, as I incorporated breathing techniques with every exercise. You will fill up with oxygen and get a total relaxation too, since I wanted this simple program to give you a chance for a better connection with yourself.

So why does the face get the "droopy" appearance as time passes? Since people don't use the face muscles, and there are 50 different muscles in your face, they tend to lose elasticity and flexibility and your appearance starts to look older. There is no rule, when this process starts to happen, it's very individual. But it's never too late to start practicing Face Yoga, or even too soon!

Face Yoga includes all areas of the face so we will combat "crow's feet", double chin, sagging jowls, under-eye bags and toning of the cheek area. This is so easy and fun you can do these exercises any time of the day. There is no equipment that you need or special place, and that is also one of the benefits.

My program also includes in several exercises the special pressure points called *meridians*. To keep it really simple, meridians are energy centers, that if correctly pressed, make optimal energy flow through our system. I included also a visualization and affirmation program to go with the exercises in order to fasten and boost the whole process. I ensure you that your feelings will be more positive and calm regarding your self-image.

For even better results I would advise you to try Yoga, Pilates or some other exercise system that will add to your general health. The programs will work perfectly together as it will reduce stress and even effect the quality of your night's sleep, and these are all factors that add up to the aging process.

So I'm actually encouraging you to change your lifestyle step by step, so you can improve the overall result of your effort.

I know it's not easy to make big changes very quickly, but as you start doing this Yoga practice, the ideas how to improve your health and looks will start coming daily. Just keep it simple, exercise for at least 10 minutes daily and everything will fall into place!

3 THE EYES

Beauty in things exists in the mind which contemplates them. ~ David Hume

Puffy eyes

First position

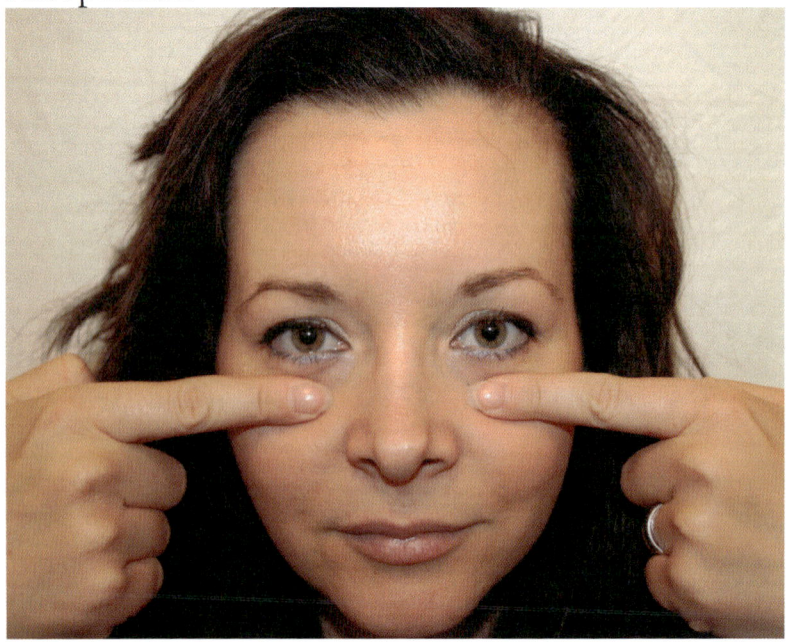

Gently press with the tips of your fingers the two pressure points as shown on the picture above. Make sure that the pressure is in the bone area and that it's not too hard. Slowly inhale and start moving your fingers to the outer eye area following the bone.

Visualization: as you inhale visualize a sparkling white light entering your entire body giving you health and beauty.

Affirmation: "Thank you for my everlasting youthful and healthy look!"

Second position:

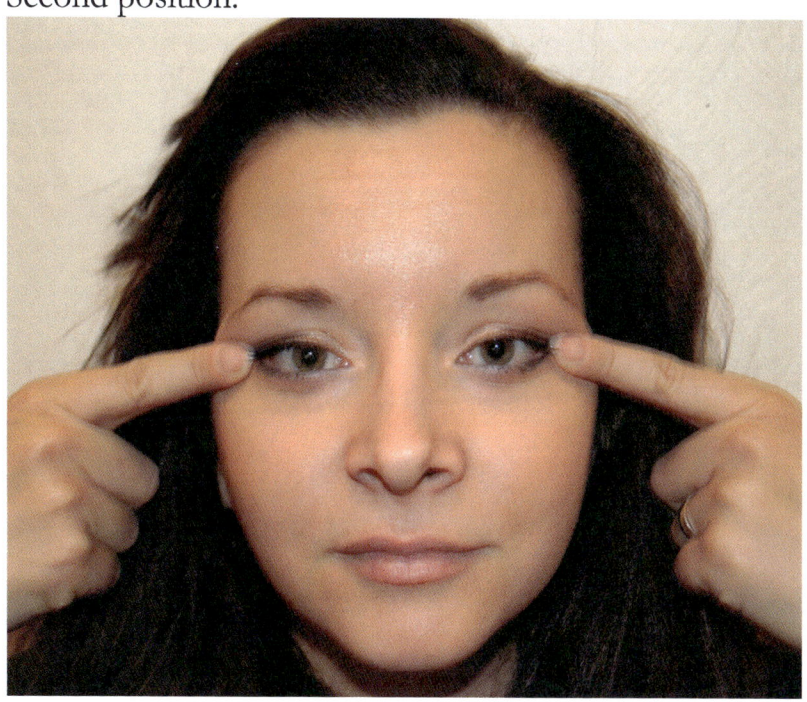

At this point you stop circling around your eyes. This point and the starting point as well are the meridians and should be treated gently. Once you reach this point exhale deeply and relax. For best results do this exercise for at least one minute a day. Results will be visible within a few days because it's highly effective against puffy eyes and the saggy skin beneath them.

Crow's Feet

Crow's feet usually appear as the result of repetitive motions when you smile or quint. They begin to form on the outside corners of your eyes usually in the mid-twenties but it also depends on the way you treat your skin every day. They may appear even a lot later if you moisturize your skin and drink a lot of water. But either way, this is a very good exercise as a prevention from as well as a cure for crow's feet.

Position number one

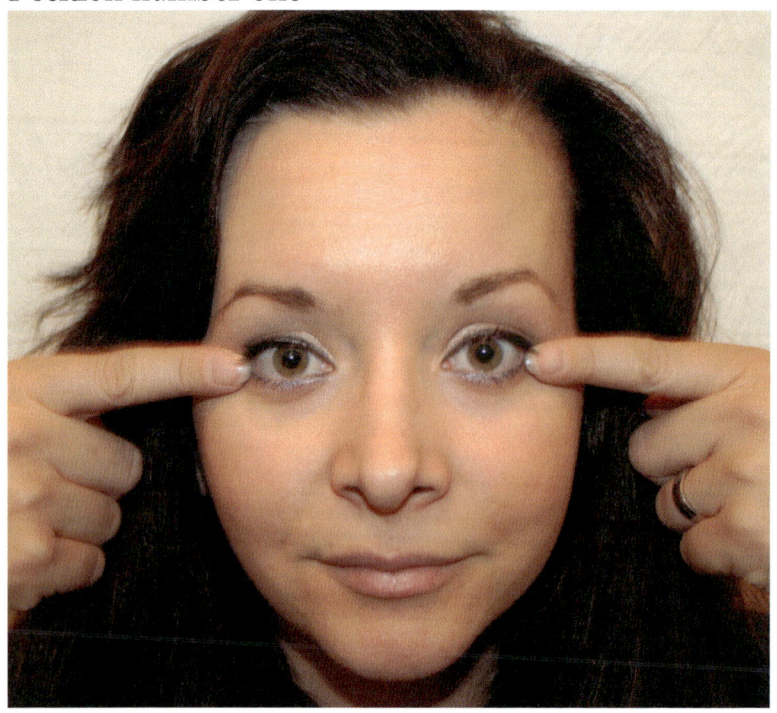

Apply gentle pressure on the outside corners of your eyes using the tips of your fingers. As you inhale, start circling around the pressure point, and as you finish the circle, exhale. Make sure that the circle is anti-clockwise and repeat the process for at least a minute daily.

Visualization: as you focus on your breathing imagine yourself like you do maybe in your fantasy versions of yourself, having the body you want and your overall ideal appearance.

Affirmation: "I love and accept my body the way it is now!"

Eyebrow fitness

This exercise will strengthen the muscles around your eyes and reduce the puffiness beneath them. It's very effective and the results increase throughout a few weeks of everyday practice.
Position number one

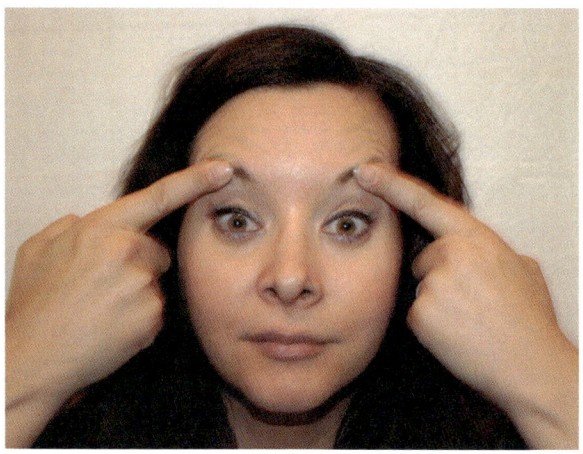

Apply pressure to the points as shown in the picture above, firmly holding eyelids from closing. As you do this position inhale deeply.

Position number two

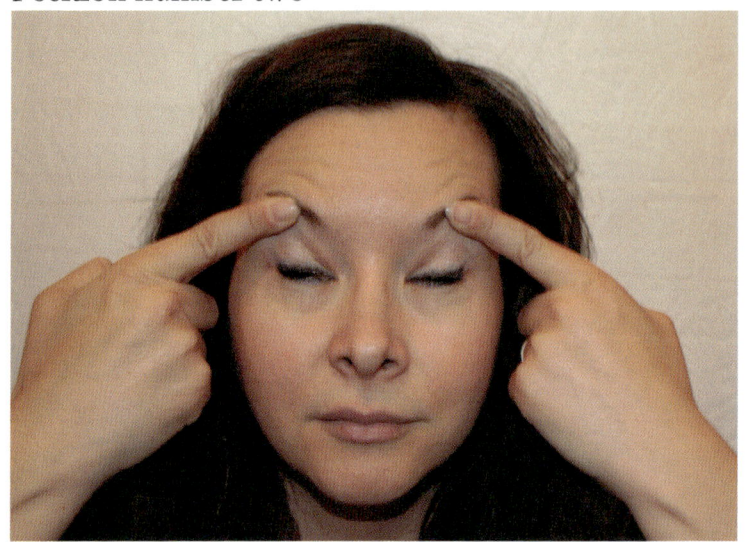

While still firmly holding the point beneath your eyebrows try to close the eyelids. You are doing the exercise correctly if you feel pressure in the eye muscles as you keep on trying to close the eyes. Do this exercise at least for a minute, three minutes a day would be optimal.

Visualization: See yourself happy and content while looking in the mirror. Imagine your ideal self looking back from the mirror. Feel the contentment after accomplishing through your efforts a younger looking face and body!

Affirmation: "Every day I look younger and more attractive", "I look beautiful and young effortlessly and I give thanks for all my blessings!"

Looking up

This exercise is very powerful and gives instant relief against eye puffiness. It helps instantly even with the worst cases. After a bad *sinusitis* I had every morning visible puffiness beneath the eyes and make up would even make things worse! This exercise was the only instant help that I found, and through time, swelling disappeared forever.

Position number one

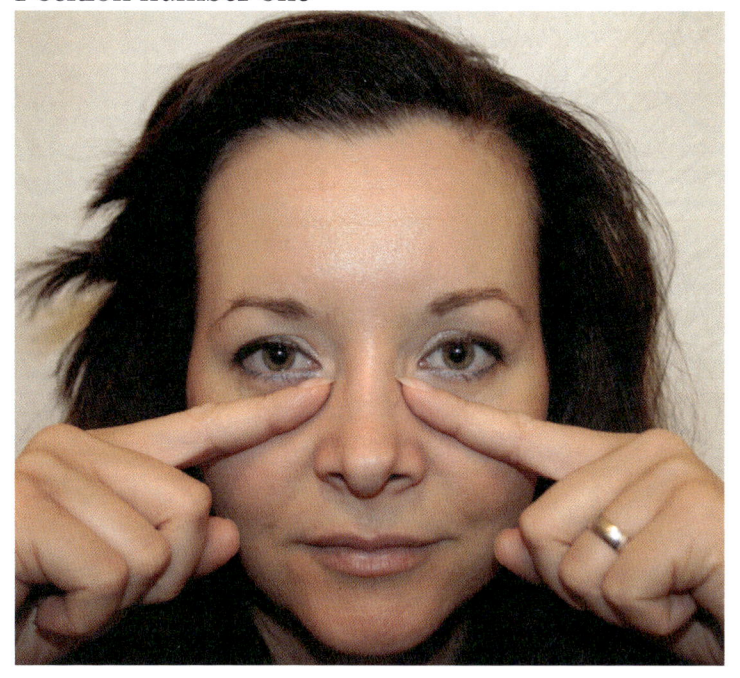

Place your forefingers as shown in the picture above. Apply a little bit stronger pressure and breath in deeply. Make sure that the pressure and position of the fingers are comfortable as they should stay like this during the whole exercise.

Position number two

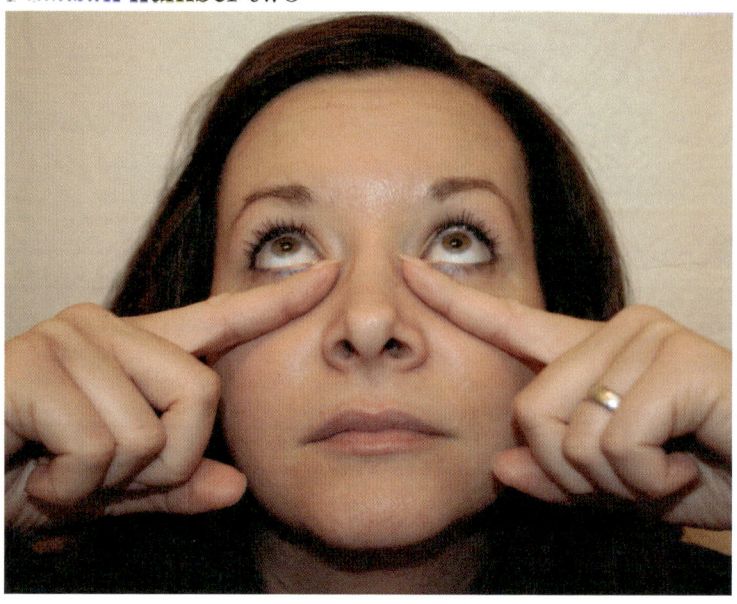

Breath normally and look up at the highest point you can and keep on looking for 30 seconds. At the beginning it was hard for me to hold 30 seconds, but I was holding as much as I could. Try to be patient, as this has instant effect on your eye area.

Position number three

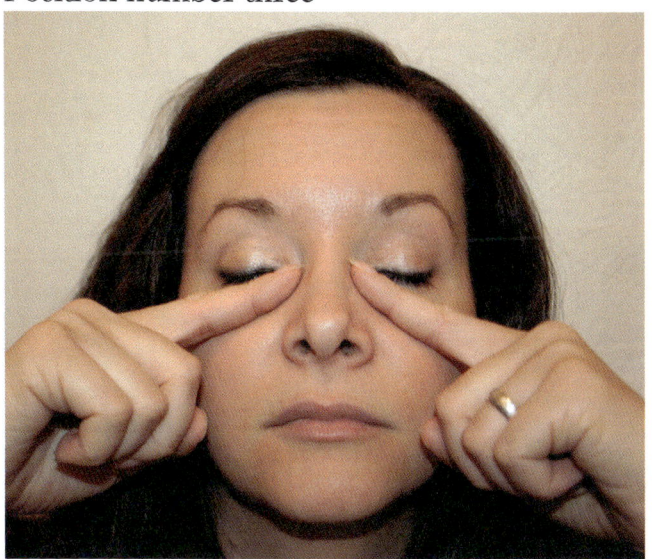

After looking up for 30 seconds take a deep breath and exhale. Close your eyes and put away your hands. Hold for a second and open your eyes.

Visualization: Imagine people telling you what beautiful eyes and skin you have. They approach you and give you many compliments. If there is something bothering you about your body, imagine that they are giving you compliments about that exact part of your body.

Affirmation: " My skin is more beautiful and radiant every day! I give thanks for my health and beauty."
"I'm so happy within my body, I keep my ideal body weight and health effortlessly!"

Wink

This exercise is very important because it strengthens the muscles around the eyes.

Position number one

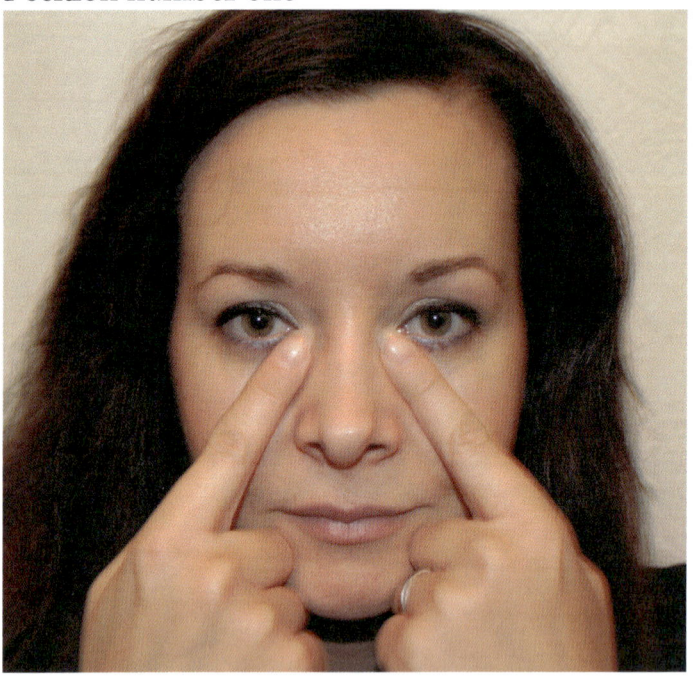

Gently press the points as shown in the picture above, and start to circle, following the bone line around the eye, all through the outer eye edges.

Position number two

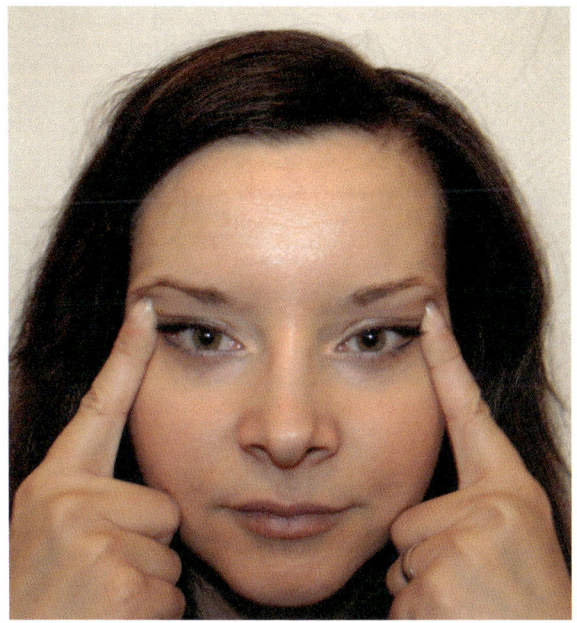

Hold very firmly these points as shown on the picture above, because the fingers must hold the resistance.

Position number three

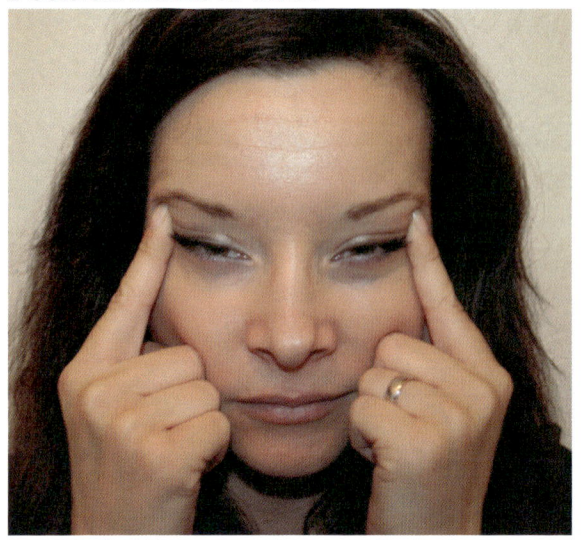

Now try to wink. If you are doing it right, there is going to be some resistance. Keep on doing it for at least a minute.

Visualization: imagine while you're doing this exercise the ideal face you want to have, try to concentrate on details.

Affirmation: "My skin is firm and radiant! I'm so happy and content with my looks!"

Eyebrows

This is very good exercise for the eyebrows and the forehead area, and is highly effective against wrinkles.

Position number one

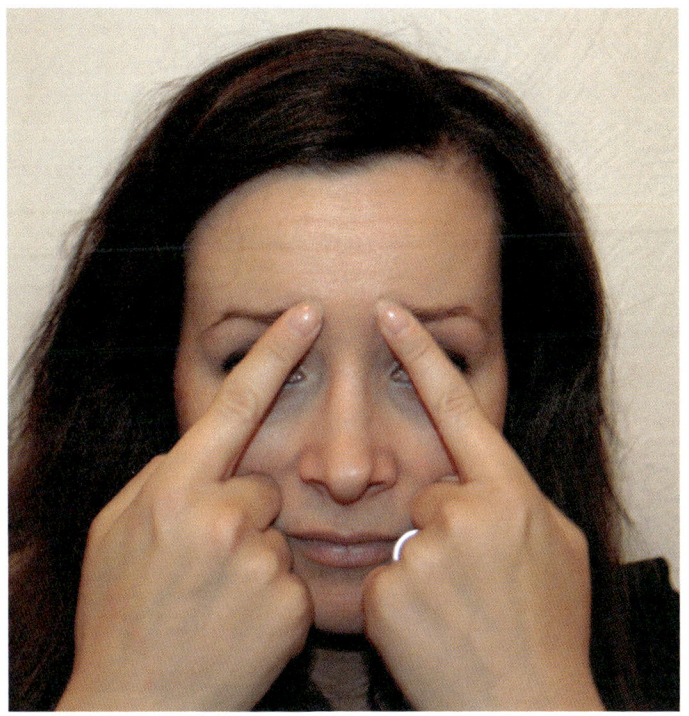

With your index finger hold the inner corner of your eyebrows, gently pull your skin and follow the eyebrow line and hold the tension while ending on the outer edges.

Position number two

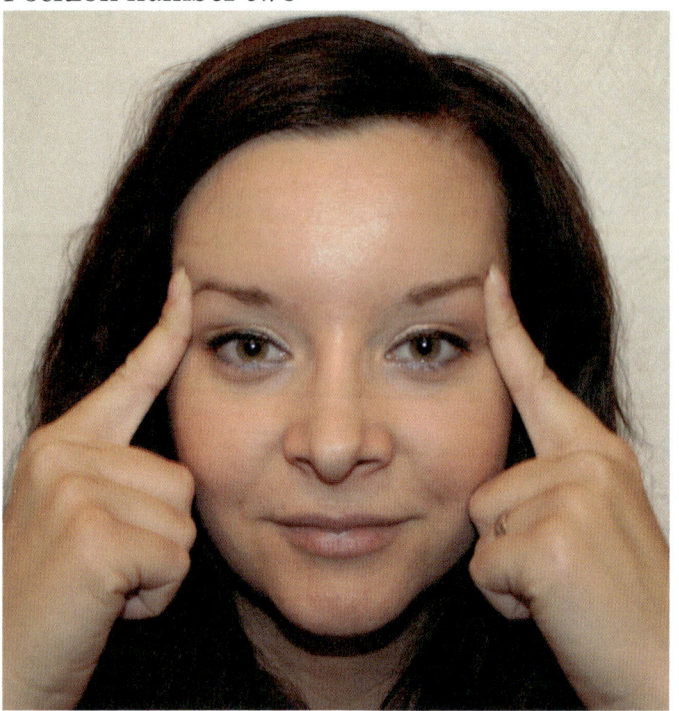

You should hold the tension on this pressure points for about 10 seconds. During the whole exercise breathe deeply and concentrate. Try to repeat the whole exercise at least 6 times.

Visualization: Imagine white sparkling light coming out of the starting points in this exercise, and visualize this light following your motion to the outer edges of your eyebrows.

Affirmation: "Wonderful healing energy is now revitalizing my skin and my face at the cellular level!"

4 FACE AND NECK EXERCISES

Pinching

This exercise is great for the whole face as it brings the circulation to your whole face area. By doing this exercise your face will have a lovely rose glow, and the blood flow will bring the nutrients to the skin. After just a few weeks (of everyday exercise), you will tone your skin so perfectly, that there will be noticeable progress to all people around you.

Position number one

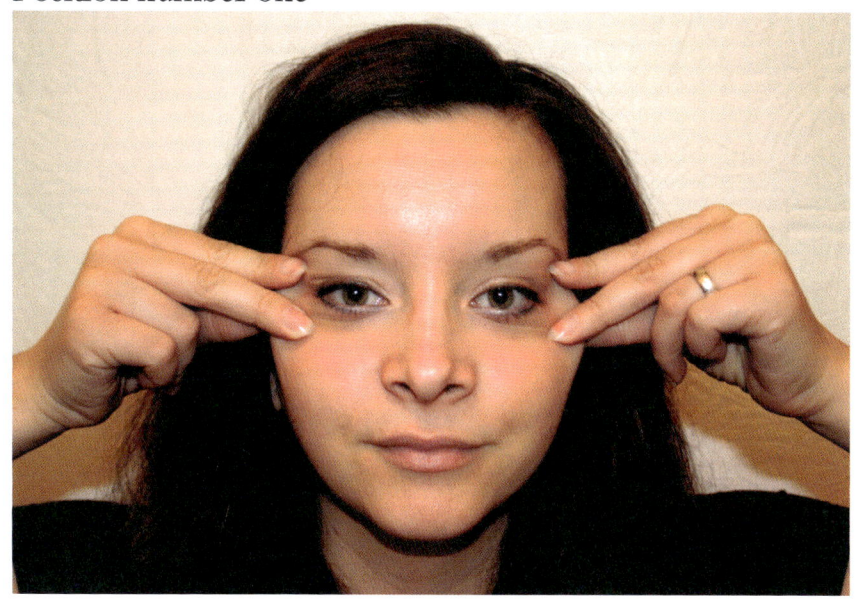

Start with the eye area. Don't pinch too hard, you must feel comfortable while doing this. Hold the position for 20 seconds, then let go. Breathe normally.

Position number two

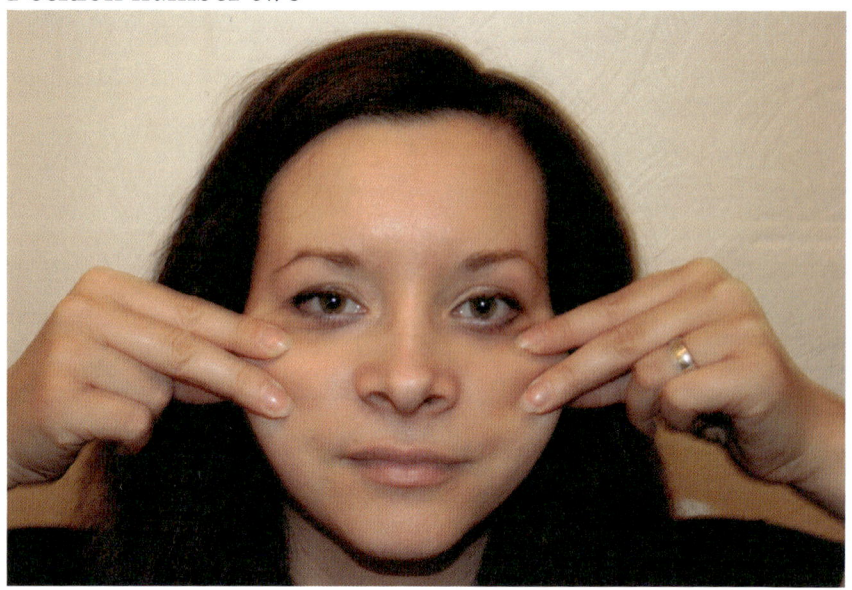

Pinch the cheeks, but again make sure that you feel comfortable. Don't pinch too hard. Hold the position for 20 seconds.

Position number three

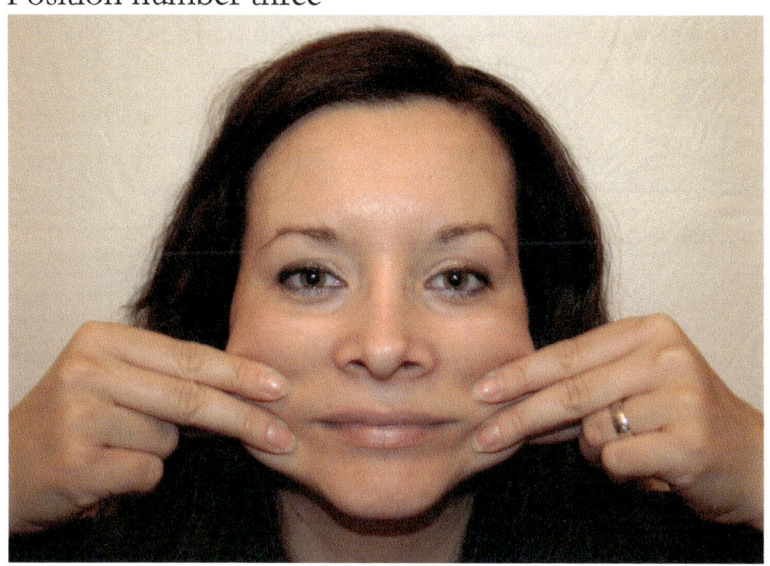

Pinch the lower part of your face and as before hold it for 20 seconds. While exercising breathe normally the whole time, and try to relax. Repeat the whole exercise three times.

Visualization: while holding your skin for 20 seconds, imagine sparkling white light filling your skin and radiating through it.

Affirmation: "Every day I look younger and more radiant."

Forehead anti-wrinkle exercise

Very effective exercise for removing the forehead wrinkles and it is relaxing too!

Position number one

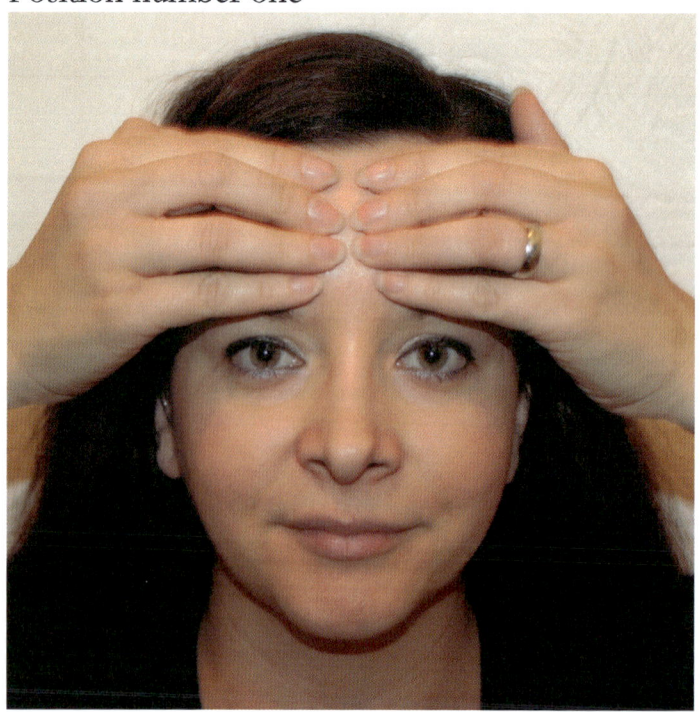

Put your fingers at the middle of your forehead and sweep them gently in a single outward motion.

Position number two

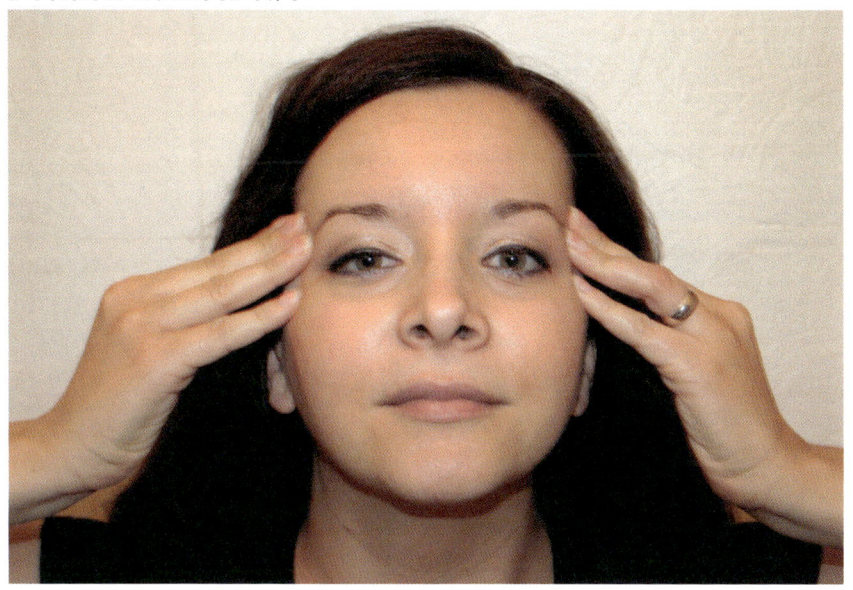

Do this exercise 6 times, and breath in at position number one, and breathe out at the position number two.

Visualization: imagine your forehead filling up with revitalizing, sparkling energy, following your motion to the edges.
Affirmation: "Revitalizing energy is healing my skin, giving me the ideal look I always wanted!"

Kissing the ceiling

This exercise is fabulous for neck and mouth both, it gives them firmness and a younger appearance! It's so easy and fun!

Position number one

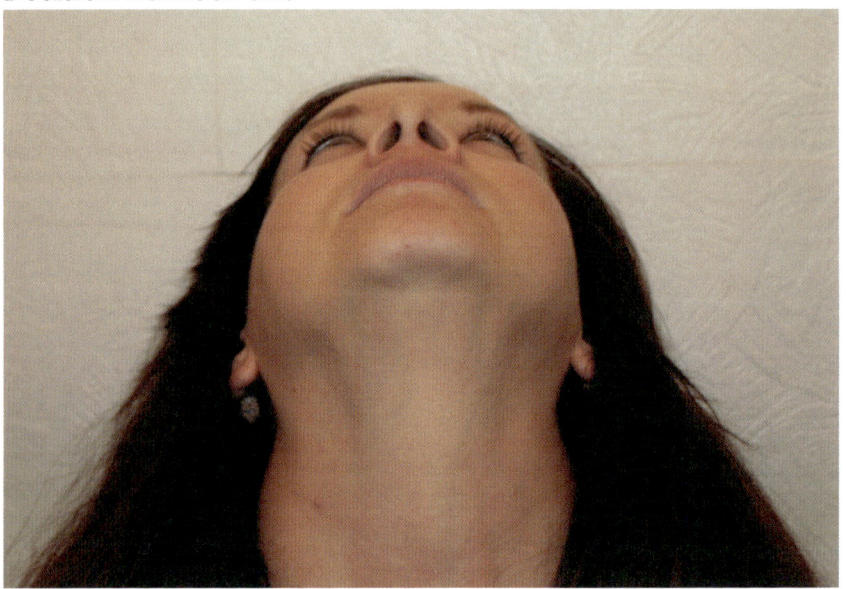

Look up as high as you can up to face the ceiling. Try to breathe normally and relax. If you feel a little pain, it's ok, that means that the exercise is working. At first this exercise seemed a little bit hard and I wouldn't be able to hold the position long enough, but with time and practice I got comfortable in this position. It really works like magic with exterminating problems like a double chin, loose skin on the neck area and even your lips will in few weeks get fuller and sexier in few weeks.

Position number two

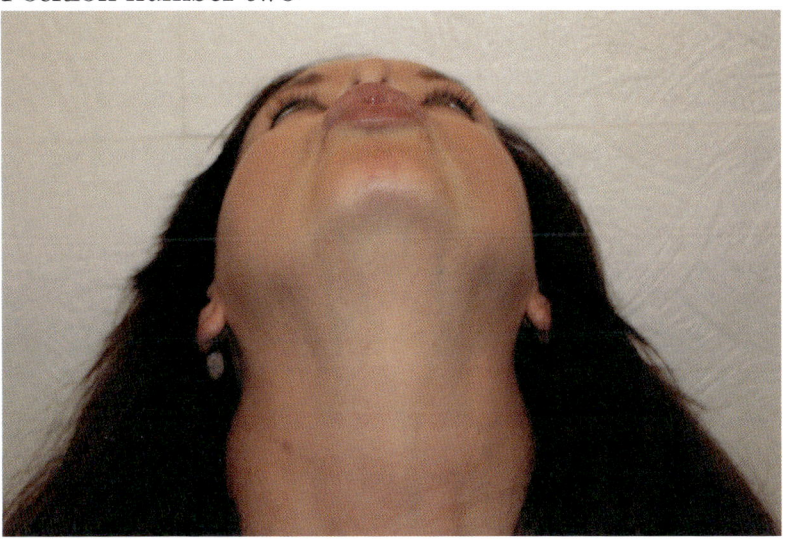

Breathe calmly and deeply through the nose and holding the position blow kisses to the ceiling. The resistance you feel during the exercise will be very strong, but for best results keep doing it for at least 30 seconds. Repeat the whole procedure 3 times.

Visualization: visualize your new and improved neck just as you wanted it always, imagine your lips full and with a sensual rosy glow…
Affirmation: "I'm so happy, I manifested all my dreams about my perfect look!"

Beautiful neck

This great exercise will "de-age" your neck in just four weeks. It's very intense, and as the previous one, will need some little adjustments. But don't give up! The benefits you get out of your efforts are countless!

Position number one

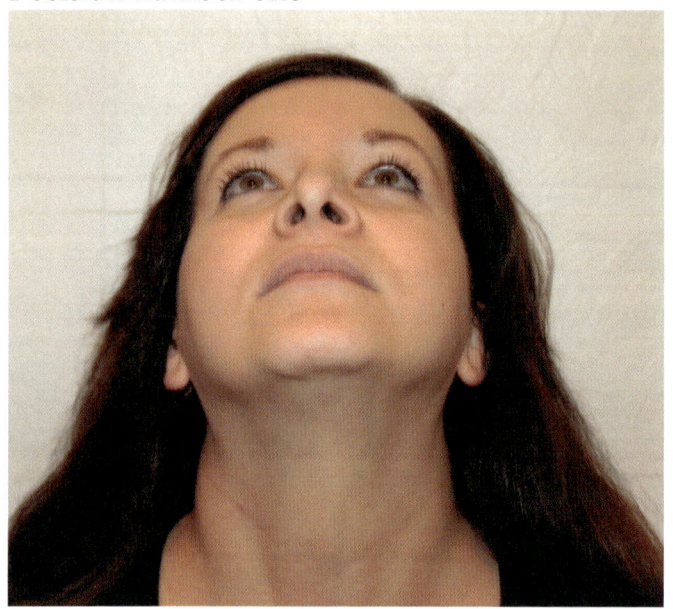

Take a deep breath and lift your head so you face the ceiling. Do it with the maximum effort, so do the stretching part correctly. Hold positions 2 and 3 each for 15 seconds. Do the exercise at least 3 times in a row for best results.

Position number two

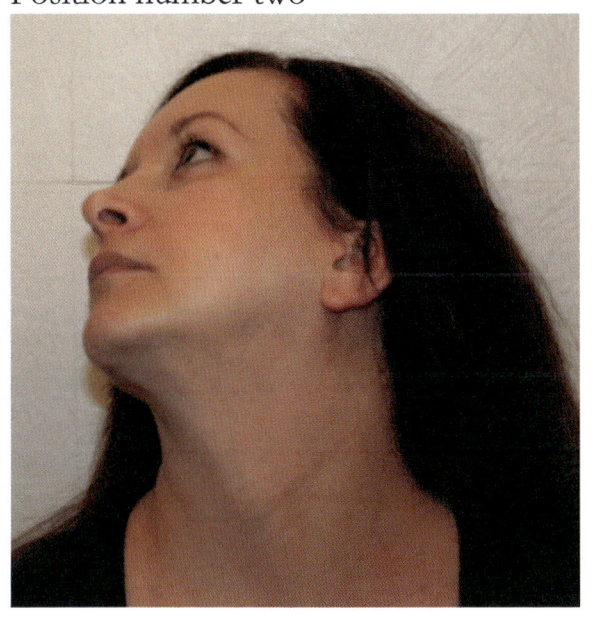

As you exhale, turn your head to the left but still holding your head as much as you can facing the ceiling.

Position number three

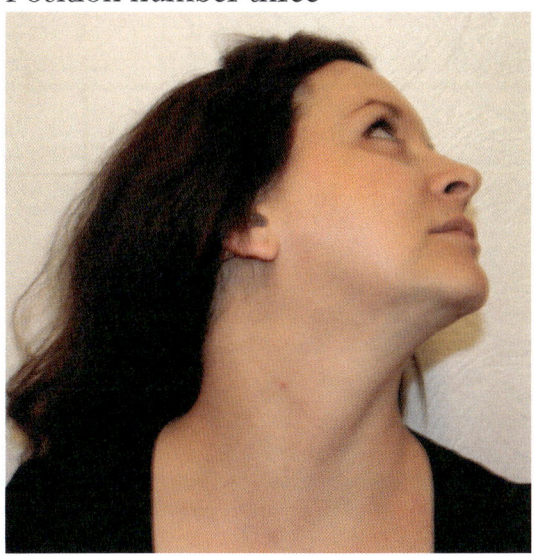

As you breathe in, slowly turn your head to the right and hold the position again for 15 seconds.

Visualization: visualize yourself in a beautiful dress (of whatever piece of clothing you prefer if you are male) that shows your slim neck and enjoy it as people comment on how young you are looking.

Affirmation: "Everything I do contributes to my overall health and beauty!"

5 WORK OUT!

I decided just before making this booklet not to write too much about theory, just as I did with my *Ultimate Balance* book. The reason for this can be found in countless books on facial exercises and yoga that include not so many exercises and explanations, but hundreds of pages of numerous theories on aging. To be honest, all of that makes me weary and bored. When I encounter a problem, I don't have time to dwell upon a possible cause and analysis, because my spiritual work has thought me better. I now try to find a solution, I don't spend my precious time on useless theories on what would or should have been. So this book is exactly what I would want to find when searching for useful practice regarding Face Yoga. Exercises and simple but clear explanations of the same and as little as possible "timewasting" on theoretical approaches. So basically, when you have this booklet in your hand, there is absolutely no excuse any more why you should not start today!
Enjoy
The Author

ABOUT THE AUTHOR

Joan Carter was born on July 16th, 1978 and is currently living and studying in Europe, finishing her PhD. Although she is a historian, since her early childhood she found interest in spiritual and mystical subjects. She published scientific papers on the subject of history in many scientific, internationally recognized magazines. Her professional life led her into the finance business, where she spent years on the level of top management. But her other true profession was her dedicated spiritual work, as she persistently was seeking upon answers that are at everybody's first interest. The pursuit for a balanced and harmonic life led her to the study of ancient Egyptian and Greek mythology, Chinese traditional medicine, the occult sciences of the middle ages, creative visualization, the *Law of attraction* and the *Emotional Freedom Technique (EFT)*.

In her adolescence she was dedicated to Yoga and martial arts, so she still loves and nurtures those values found in that part of her life. In fact some of the knowledge she passed onto her daughter, that is working on some of her projects as well. Joan is happily married and lives with her family in Europe where she is preparing some more projects on spiritual subject.

Printed in Great Britain
by Amazon.co.uk, Ltd.,
Marston Gate.